THE AIP DIET FOR WEIGHT LOSS

A personalized plan for using the AIP Diet to lose weight and keep it off.

COPYRIGHT © 2023

All rights reserved.

The information contained in this book is based on the author's research and experience. While the author has made every effort to provide accurate and up-to-date information, errors and omissions may occur. The author and publisher assume no responsibility for any errors or omissions or for any actions taken based on the information contained in this book.

TABLE OF CONTENTS

INTRODUCTION

In a world where diets often come and go like fleeting trends, the Autoimmune Protocol (AIP) diet stands as a unique and multifaceted approach, offering far more than a mere weight loss regimen. It is a powerful tool that not only assists in shedding excess pounds but also, critically, aims to address the underlying factors contributing to weight gain while fostering sustainable and long-term health. The AIP diet is a testament to the idea that a personalized and holistic approach to nutrition can serve as a cornerstone for achieving and maintaining a healthy weight.

In the midst of the modern dietary landscape, where processed foods laden with hidden sugars and inflammatory agents have become the norm, the prevalence of obesity and associated chronic health conditions has reached staggering proportions. Traditional diets often revolve around the rudimentary concept of calorie counting, often overlooking the intricate relationships between food, our immune system, and overall well-being. In contrast, the AIP diet sets forth a more comprehensive and insightful perspective by emphasizing the elimination of foods known to trigger inflammation and immune system responses within the body.

As we embark on this journey through the AIP diet, we will explore how this approach transcends the realm of mere weight loss. It delves into the roots of weight gain, acknowledging that excess pounds are often symptomatic of deeper imbalances in the body. By understanding and applying the principles of the AIP diet, you will not only be equipped to shed unwanted weight but will also embark on a profound transformation towards a healthier, more vitalized existence.

This comprehensive guide will unveil the intricacies of the AIP diet, equipping you with the knowledge and tools necessary to craft a personalized plan that aligns with your unique circumstances and aspirations. Whether you are grappling with persistent weight issues, navigating the challenges of autoimmune conditions, or simply striving for a more wholesome lifestyle, the AIP diet offers a beacon of hope. It promises not only the potential for weight loss but also the attainment of enduring health and vitality.

In the pages that follow, we will delve into the nuanced facets of the AIP diet, demonstrating how it can serve as a catalyst for shedding excess weight and nurturing a lasting sense of well-being. Together, we will explore the dictary choices, lifestyle adjustments, and mindful approaches that can empower you to achieve your weight loss goals and, equally importantly, sustain them for the long term. So, let us embark on this transformative journey through the world of the Autoimmune Protocol diet, where the pursuit of a healthy weight becomes synonymous with the cultivation of a richer, more balanced life.

CHAPTER ONE

WHAT IS THE AIP DIET AND ITS ORIGINS?

The Autoimmune Protocol (AIP) diet, sometimes referred to as the Autoimmune Paleo diet, is a specialized dietary approach designed to help individuals manage autoimmune diseases and related health conditions. It is a stricter variation of the paleo diet that focuses on reducing inflammation and promoting gut health. The AIP diet aims to alleviate autoimmune symptoms, such as joint pain, fatigue, and digestive issues, by eliminating potentially inflammatory foods and incorporating nutrient-dense, healing foods.

Origins of the AIP Diet:

The AIP diet can trace its origins back to the paleo diet, which is based on the idea of eating like our prehistoric ancestors. The paleo diet emphasizes whole, unprocessed foods and excludes grains, dairy, legumes, processed sugars, and many other modern foods that are believed to contribute to inflammation and various health issues.

The AIP diet evolved from the paleo diet in the early 2010s, primarily through the work of two prominent autoimmune advocates and authors, Dr. Sarah Ballantyne and Mickey Trescott:

• Dr. Sarah Ballantyne (Ph.D.): Dr. Ballantyne, a medical biophysicist and author, is credited with popularizing the AIP diet. She published "The Paleo Approach: Reverse Autoimmune Disease and Heal Your Body" in 2014. This comprehensive book outlined the scientific basis for the AIP diet and provided practical guidance for individuals with autoimmune conditions.

• Mickey Trescott: Mickey Trescott, a chef and author, further popularized the AIP diet with her book "The Autoimmune Paleo Cookbook" published in 2016. Her cookbook offered a wide range of AIP-compliant recipes, making it easier for people to follow the diet while enjoying flavorful meals.

Key Principles of the AIP Diet:

The AIP diet focuses on the following key principles:

• Elimination of Inflammatory Foods: The AIP diet eliminates common trigger foods that may contribute to inflammation, such as grains, dairy, legumes, processed sugars, nightshade vegetables, eggs, nuts, and seeds.

• Emphasis on Nutrient-Dense Foods: AIP encourages the consumption of nutrient-dense foods like grass-fed meats, wild-caught fish, organ meats, non-starchy vegetables, healthy fats (e.g., coconut oil, olive oil, and avocado), and some fruits (in moderation).

• Gut Health: AIP places a strong emphasis on healing the gut, as it is believed to play a crucial role in autoimmune conditions. Probiotic-rich foods and bone broth are often recommended to support gut health.

• Lifestyle Factors: Beyond diet, AIP also addresses lifestyle factors like sleep, stress management, and regular physical activity as essential components of overall well-being.

• Gradual Reintroduction: After a period of strict elimination, some individuals may reintroduce certain foods one at a time to identify specific triggers and gauge their tolerance.

The AIP diet is highly individualized, and people with autoimmune conditions often work closely with healthcare professionals or registered dietitians to tailor the approach to their specific needs and monitor their progress. While the AIP diet is primarily designed to manage autoimmune diseases, some individuals have found it helpful for weight loss and general health improvement when applied mindfully.

WHAT IS WEIGHT LOSS?

Weight loss refers to the reduction in body weight, typically as a result of a deliberate effort to decrease excess body fat or overall body mass. It can occur for various reasons, including improving overall health, managing specific medical conditions, enhancing physical appearance, or achieving specific fitness goals.

Weight loss can occur through a combination of factors, including changes in diet, increased physical activity, and modifications to lifestyle habits. It is often measured in terms of pounds or kilograms lost and is typically tracked over a specific period, such as weeks or months.

Weight loss can have both positive and negative effects on an individual's health, depending on the approach taken, the amount of weight lost, and the overall context. Healthy and sustainable weight loss is generally associated with benefits such as:

• Improved Health: Weight loss, especially when it involves reducing excess body fat, can lower the risk of various chronic health conditions, including heart disease, type 2 diabetes, and certain types of cancer.

• Increased Energy Levels: Shedding excess weight can lead to increased energy and improved mobility, making it easier to engage in physical activities.

• Enhanced Self-Esteem: Achieving weight loss goals can boost self-confidence and improve self-esteem, positively impacting mental health and overall well-being.

• Better Physical Function: Weight loss can lead to improved physical function, reduced joint pain, and increased mobility, especially in individuals who were previously overweight or obese.

• Management of Medical Conditions: Weight loss is often recommended as a part of the management plan for conditions like obesity, sleep apnea, and high blood pressure.

However, it's important to note that extreme or rapid weight loss, especially through unhealthy or unsustainable methods, can have negative consequences on health, such as muscle loss, nutrient deficiencies, and potential negative impacts on metabolism. Crash diets, extreme caloric restriction, or excessive exercise can be harmful and are generally discouraged.

A healthy approach to weight loss involves gradual and sustainable changes to diet and lifestyle, along with regular physical activity. It should also consider individual needs, goals, and overall health status. Consulting with a healthcare professional or registered dietitian is often advisable when embarking on a weight loss journey to ensure that it is done safely and effectively. Additionally, long-term maintenance of a healthy weight is often more important than just achieving a temporary reduction in weight.

HOW TO PREPARE TO START THE AIP DIET

Preparing to start the Autoimmune Protocol (AIP) diet requires careful planning and a commitment to making significant dietary and lifestyle changes. Here are the steps to help you prepare effectively:

• Educate Yourself: Begin by thoroughly researching the AIP diet. Read books, articles, and reputable online sources to understand the principles, allowed foods, and those to be eliminated. Familiarize yourself with the core concepts and rationale behind the diet.

• Consult with a Healthcare Professional: Before starting the AIP diet, consult with a healthcare professional, preferably a registered dietitian or a healthcare provider familiar with autoimmune conditions. They can assess your individual health needs, provide personalized guidance, and ensure that the AIP diet is appropriate for your specific situation.

• Identify Your Triggers and Goals: Determine the autoimmune condition or health issues you're seeking to address with the AIP diet. Identify any specific food triggers or symptoms that you want to alleviate. Set clear and realistic health goals for yourself to track your progress.

• Kitchen Cleanup: Clean out your kitchen to remove all non-AIP-compliant foods and ingredients. This will reduce temptation and make it easier to adhere to the diet. Check labels carefully, as many processed foods contain hidden ingredients that are not AIP-friendly.

• Meal Planning: Plan your meals in advance. Create a list of AIP-compliant recipes, and consider batch cooking and meal prep to save time during the week. Stock up on AIP-approved ingredients such as grass-fed meats, wild-caught fish, non-starchy vegetables, and healthy fats.

• Create a Shopping List: Prepare a detailed shopping list based on your planned AIP meals. Ensure you have all the necessary ingredients, so you're less likely to resort to non-compliant foods out of convenience.

• Explore AIP-Friendly Recipes: Gather a collection of AIP-friendly recipes that you find appealing and diverse. Having a variety of recipes will help you stay motivated and prevent dietary boredom.

• Meal Replacements and Snacks: Identify AIP-compliant snacks and meal replacement options for times when you need quick and convenient food choices. Fresh fruits, vegetables, homemade jerky, or AIP-friendly snack bars can be good options.

• Support System: Inform friends and family of your dietary changes, and seek their understanding and support. Consider joining AIP online communities or support groups to connect with others who are following the same diet for guidance and motivation.

• Learn to Read Labels: Familiarize yourself with ingredient labels on packaged foods. Be vigilant about avoiding hidden non-compliant ingredients, such as certain additives, preservatives, and flavorings.

• Experiment with Reintroductions (Later): While the initial phase of the AIP diet is strict, remember that it's not meant to be followed indefinitely. Eventually, you may reintroduce eliminated foods one at a time to assess your tolerance. Consult with your healthcare provider for guidance on this phase.

• Manage Stress and Lifestyle Factors: Prioritize stress management techniques like meditation, yoga, or deep breathing exercises, as stress can exacerbate autoimmune symptoms. Ensure you're getting adequate sleep and incorporate regular physical activity into your routine.

Remember that the AIP diet can be challenging, and it may take time to adjust to the new way of eating. Be patient with yourself and stay committed to your health goals. It's also important to monitor your progress and make adjustments as needed with the guidance of a healthcare professional.

HOW TO LOSE WEIGHT WITH THE AIP DIET

Losing weight with the Autoimmune Protocol (AIP) diet involves adapting the principles of the AIP to focus on weight loss while still managing autoimmune symptoms and promoting overall health. Here's a step-by-step guide on how to approach weight loss with the AIP diet:

• Consult with a Healthcare Professional: Before starting any weight loss plan, especially one as restrictive as the AIP diet, consult with a healthcare professional or registered dietitian. They can help you create a personalized plan that considers your specific health needs and goals.

• Understand AIP Principles: Educate yourself about the core principles of the AIP diet, which include eliminating foods that may trigger inflammation and immune reactions while emphasizing nutrient-dense, healing foods.

• Set Realistic Weight Loss Goals: Define your weight loss goals. Make them specific, measurable, achievable, relevant, and time-bound (SMART). For example, "Lose 1-2 pounds per week and improve autoimmune symptoms."

• Plan AIP-Compliant Meals: Create a meal plan that adheres to the AIP guidelines but focuses on weight loss. Your meals should include a balance of AIP-approved foods, such as:

1. Lean proteins: Grass-fed meats, wild-caught fish, and organ meats.

2. Non-starchy vegetables: Leafy greens, cruciferous vegetables, and other non-nightshade varieties.

3. Healthy fats: Coconut oil, olive oil, avocado, and fatty fish.

4. Fruits (in moderation): Berries, apples, and pears.

5. Herbs and spices: Ginger, turmeric, oregano, and others.

• Control Portion Sizes: While the AIP diet doesn't require strict calorie counting, be mindful of portion sizes, especially for calorie-dense foods like fats and proteins. Portion control can help with weight management.

• Limit High-Calorie AIP Foods: Be cautious with foods like nuts, seeds, and coconut products, which can be caloric-dense. Consume them in moderation, especially if weight loss is your goal.

• Stay Hydrated: Drink plenty of water throughout the day to support digestion and metabolism. Sometimes, thirst can be mistaken for hunger.

• Monitor Your Intake: Keep a food journal to track your meals, portion sizes, and any emotional or environmental triggers for eating. This can help you identify patterns and areas for improvement.

• Include Regular Physical Activity: Incorporate regular exercise into your routine. Consult with a fitness professional to create a balanced workout plan that aligns with your AIP goals and fitness level.

• Prioritize Sleep and Stress Management: Aim for 7-9 hours of quality sleep each night, as inadequate sleep can hinder weight loss efforts. Practice stress management techniques such as meditation, yoga, or deep breathing exercises to reduce stress-related eating.

• Monitor Progress and Adjustments: Regularly assess your weight loss progress and overall well-being. Adjust your meal plan and exercise routine as needed based on your goals and how your body responds.

• Seek Support: Join AIP online communities or support groups to connect with others following the AIP diet for weight loss. Sharing experiences and tips can be motivating and helpful.

Remember that weight loss on the AIP diet, like any other diet, takes time and commitment. Prioritize overall health and well-being, and consult with a healthcare professional or dietitian to ensure that your approach is safe and effective for your specific needs and goals.

AIP DIET PHASES

The Autoimmune Protocol (AIP) diet is often divided into several phases to help individuals manage autoimmune conditions, identify food sensitivities, and gradually reintroduce eliminated foods. While the specific phase names and duration can vary, here's a general outline of the typical phases of the AIP diet:

Elimination Phase:

• Duration: Generally, 30 days or longer, depending on individual needs and symptoms.

• Objective: The initial phase involves the strict elimination of foods that are commonly known to trigger inflammation and autoimmune reactions. These foods include grains, dairy, legumes, processed sugars, nightshade vegetables, eggs, nuts, and seeds.

• Allowed Foods: Focus on nutrient-dense foods such as grass-fed meats, wild-caught fish, organ meats, non-starchy vegetables, healthy fats (coconut oil, olive oil, avocado), and some fruits (in moderation).

• Lifestyle Factors: Stress management, sleep, and physical activity are also emphasized during this phase to support overall well-being.

Healing Phase:

• Duration: Ongoing, as the healing phase is an integral part of the AIP diet.

• Objective: This phase continues the strict elimination of trigger foods while concentrating on nourishing the body with nutrient-dense foods that support gut health and reduce inflammation. The emphasis is on healing the gut, which is often a key factor in autoimmune conditions.

• Allowed Foods: The same foods allowed in the elimination phase, with a focus on bone broth, fermented foods, and probiotics to support gut health.

Reintroduction Phase:

• Duration: Variable, depending on individual progress and goals.

• Objective: The reintroduction phase involves systematically reintroducing eliminated foods one at a time to assess individual tolerance and identify triggers. This phase helps individuals determine which foods they can safely incorporate back into their diet without causing autoimmune symptoms.

• Method: Foods are reintroduced gradually, starting with those considered less likely to trigger reactions (e.g., eggs) and progressing to more potentially problematic foods (e.g., nightshades).

• Monitoring: Carefully monitor symptoms and reactions during this phase. Keep a food journal to track how each reintroduced food affects your body.

Maintenance Phase:

• Duration: Ongoing.

• Objective: After identifying trigger foods and establishing a personalized set of tolerated foods, individuals enter the maintenance phase. In this phase, the goal is to maintain a diet that supports both autoimmune management and overall health.

• Allowed Foods: Continue to emphasize AIP-compliant foods while incorporating reintroduced foods that are well-tolerated.

• Lifestyle Factors: Stress management, quality sleep, and regular physical activity remain important components of the maintenance phase to sustain health and well-being.

It's crucial to remember that the AIP diet should be personalized based on your specific health needs, symptoms, and goals. Some individuals may need to remain in the elimination phase for an extended period, while others may successfully reintroduce a wider variety of foods relatively quickly. Consulting with a healthcare professional or registered dietitian experienced in the AIP diet can help you navigate these phases effectively and ensure that the approach is tailored to your individual circumstances.

AIP-COMPLIANT FOODS

The Autoimmune Protocol (AIP) diet focuses on eliminating foods that may trigger inflammation and autoimmune reactions while emphasizing nutrient-dense, healing foods. Below is a comprehensive list of AIP-compliant foods that you can include in your diet:

Proteins:

• Grass-fed and pasture-raised meats (beef, lamb, pork, poultry)

• Wild-caught fish (salmon, mackerel, sardines, etc.)

- Organ meats (liver, heart, kidneys)

- Game meats (venison, bison, etc.)

- Gelatin (from grass-fed sources)

Vegetables (Non-Starchy):

- Leafy greens (spinach, kale, collard greens, arugula, etc.)

- Cruciferous vegetables (broccoli, cauliflower, cabbage, Brussels sprouts)

- Root vegetables (sweet potatoes, carrots, beets, turnips, rutabaga)

- Squash (acorn, butternut, spaghetti squash, etc.)

- Artichokes

- Asparagus

- Mushrooms

- Zucchini

- Onions (excluding seed-based spices)

• Garlic

Fruits (in Moderation):

• Apples

• Berries (blueberries, strawberries, raspberries, etc.)

• Pears

• Avocado

• Coconut (fresh, coconut oil, coconut milk)

• Fresh figs (in moderation)

Healthy Fats:

• Coconut oil

• Olive oil (extra-virgin)

• Avocado oil

• Rendered animal fats (lard, tallow, duck fat)

Herbs and Spices (Non-Seed-Based):

• Turmeric

- Ginger

- Oregano

- Thyme

- Basil

- Mint

- Cilantro

- Rosemary

- Sage

Beverages:

- Bone broth (homemade, without non-compliant ingredients)

- Herbal teas (chamomile, mint, ginger, etc.)

- Coconut water (in moderation)

- Filtered water

Condiments and Flavorings (Homemade):

- Apple cider vinegar

• Coconut aminos (a soy sauce substitute)

• Homemade dressings and sauces using compliant ingredients

• Herbs, spices, and seasonings (non-seed-based)

Nuts and Seeds (Occasional, for Some Individuals):

• Coconut (not a true nut, but often classified as one)

• Coconut products (coconut flakes, coconut butter)

• Coconut flour (used sparingly)

• Tigernuts (a type of tuber)

• Occasionally, small amounts of seed spices like mustard, cumin, and coriander if tolerated (introduce cautiously during the reintroduction phase)

Probiotic-Rich Foods (for Gut Health):

• Fermented vegetables (sauerkraut, kimchi)

• Fermented beverages (kombucha, water kefir)

- Coconut yogurt (homemade, without non-compliant ingredients)

Please note that while this list covers the basics of AIP-compliant foods, individual tolerances may vary. It's crucial to pay attention to your body's response to different foods and consult with a healthcare professional or registered dietitian experienced in the AIP diet for personalized guidance and meal planning. Additionally, during the elimination phase, it's essential to strictly avoid non-compliant foods to assess their impact on your health accurately.

THE FOODS AND SUBSTANCES TO AVOID OR LIMIT DURING THE AIP PROTOCOL

The Autoimmune Protocol (AIP) is a dietary approach designed to reduce inflammation, support the immune system, and alleviate symptoms of autoimmune conditions. To achieve these goals, it's essential to eliminate or limit certain foods and substances that are known to trigger autoimmune reactions and inflammation. Here is a detailed explanation of the foods and substances to avoid or limit during the AIP protocol:

1. Grains: Avoid all grains, including wheat, barley, rye, oats, corn, and rice. These grains contain proteins such as gluten and lectins, which can trigger inflammation and autoimmune responses.

2. Dairy: Eliminate all forms of dairy, including milk, cheese, yogurt, and butter. Dairy proteins (casein and whey) and lactose can be problematic for many individuals with autoimmune conditions.

3. Legumes: Exclude legumes such as beans, lentils, chickpeas, and peanuts. Legumes contain lectins, phytates, and other compounds that may contribute to inflammation and digestive issues.

4. Processed Sugars: Avoid all forms of processed sugars, including cane sugar, high-fructose corn syrup, and artificial sweeteners. Excess sugar consumption can lead to inflammation and negatively impact the gut microbiome.

5. Nightshade Vegetables: Limit or avoid nightshade vegetables, including tomatoes, potatoes, peppers (bell peppers, chili peppers), and eggplants. Some individuals with

autoimmune conditions may be sensitive to alkaloids found in nightshades.

6. Eggs: Exclude eggs from your diet, as they contain proteins that can trigger autoimmune reactions in some individuals. You can reintroduce eggs later during the AIP protocol to assess your tolerance.

7. Nuts and Seeds: Avoid all nuts and seeds during the elimination phase of the AIP diet, as they contain anti-nutrients and proteins that may irritate the gut. However, some individuals may reintroduce certain nuts and seeds later in moderation during the reintroduction phase.

8. Seed-Based Spices: Limit or avoid seed-based spices such as mustard seeds, cumin, and coriander during the elimination phase. These spices contain compounds that may affect individuals with autoimmune conditions. You can reintroduce them gradually during the reintroduction phase.

9. Coffee and Alcohol: Eliminate coffee and alcoholic beverages during the initial phase of the AIP protocol, as they can contribute to inflammation, disrupt sleep, and negatively affect

the gut. You can reintroduce them cautiously during the reintroduction phase, if desired.

10. Food Additives and Artificial Ingredients: Avoid food additives, artificial preservatives, colors, and flavors. Processed foods often contain these ingredients, which can be detrimental to overall health and may exacerbate autoimmune symptoms.

11. Non-Steroidal Anti-Inflammatory Drugs (NSAIDs): Limit or avoid NSAIDs like ibuprofen and aspirin, as they can exacerbate gut issues and contribute to inflammation.

12. Excessive Alcohol and Caffeine: Limit alcohol consumption to moderation, and reduce or eliminate caffeine intake, as both can impact sleep quality and exacerbate autoimmune symptoms.

It's important to note that the AIP protocol is typically implemented in stages, with strict elimination of these foods and substances during the initial phase, followed by gradual reintroductions during the reintroduction phase to determine individual tolerances. Consulting with a healthcare professional or registered dietitian experienced in the AIP diet can provide personalized guidance and help you tailor the protocol to your specific needs and health goals.

HOW TO DESIGN MEAL PLANS THAT ADHERE TO THE AIP GUIDELINES

Designing meal plans that adhere to the Autoimmune Protocol (AIP) guidelines requires careful consideration of the foods to include and avoid while ensuring that your meals are balanced, nutrient-dense, and flavorful. Here's a step-by-step guide to help you create AIP-compliant meal plans:

1. Understand AIP Guidelines: Familiarize yourself with the AIP guidelines, including foods to include and those to avoid, as outlined in previous responses.

2. Plan Your Meals: Create a weekly or monthly meal plan that includes breakfast, lunch, dinner, and snacks. Planning in advance helps you stay organized and ensures you have AIP-compliant options readily available.

3. Include Protein Sources: Prioritize high-quality protein sources, such as grass-fed meats, wild-caught fish, and organ

meats. Plan to include a protein source in each meal to support muscle maintenance and overall health.

4. Incorporate Non-Starchy Vegetables: Build your meals around non-starchy vegetables like leafy greens, broccoli, cauliflower, and carrots. These vegetables are rich in vitamins, minerals, and fiber.

5. Add Healthy Fats: Include healthy fats like coconut oil, olive oil, and avocado in your meals. These fats provide satiety and are important for nutrient absorption.

6. Select AIP-Friendly Fruits: Enjoy AIP-compliant fruits in moderation, such as berries, apples, and pears. These can be included in snacks or as part of your breakfast.

7. Use Herbs and Spices (Non-Seed-Based): Season your dishes with AIP-friendly herbs and spices like turmeric, ginger, oregano, thyme, basil, and mint for flavor without the risk of seeds or nightshades.

8. Create Balanced Meals: Aim for balanced meals that include protein, vegetables, and healthy fats. For example, a dinner might consist of grilled chicken (protein), roasted sweet

potatoes (vegetables), and a side salad with olive oil dressing (healthy fats).

9. Plan Batch Cooking: Consider batch cooking and meal prep to save time during the week. Prepare larger quantities of AIP-compliant dishes and store them in the refrigerator or freezer for convenient meals.

10. Explore AIP Recipes: Explore AIP-friendly recipes from cookbooks, websites, or AIP communities. There are many creative and delicious recipes that adhere to the guidelines, including AIP-friendly versions of classic dishes.

11. Variety and Rotation: Incorporate a variety of AIP-compliant foods to ensure you're getting a wide range of nutrients. Rotate your food choices to prevent dietary monotony.

12. Mindful Snacking: Plan for AIP-compliant snacks when needed. Options may include sliced vegetables with guacamole, homemade beef jerky, or AIP-friendly snack bars.

13. Stay Hydrated: Remember to drink plenty of water throughout the day. You can also enjoy herbal teas as AIP-compliant beverages.

14. Consider Food Intolerances: Be mindful of individual food sensitivities or allergies. If you suspect a particular food is problematic, avoid it until you can reintroduce it during the AIP reintroduction phase.

15. Record and Adjust: Keep a food journal to track your meals and how they make you feel. This can help identify any triggers or sensitivities and guide adjustments to your meal plan.

16. Seek Support and Guidance: If you're new to the AIP diet or need personalized guidance, consider consulting with a healthcare professional or registered dietitian experienced in the AIP protocol. They can help tailor your meal plan to your specific needs and goals.

Remember that the AIP diet is highly individualized, and your meal plan should align with your health objectives and dietary preferences. Creating a well-balanced and diverse menu can make following the AIP guidelines more manageable and enjoyable while supporting your overall health.

The Autoimmune Protocol (AIP) diet, initially designed to manage autoimmune diseases and reduce inflammation, can indirectly support weight loss for some individuals. While weight loss is not the primary goal of the AIP diet, several factors associated with the diet can contribute to weight management and potential weight loss:

• Improved Nutrient Density: The AIP diet emphasizes whole, nutrient-dense foods like fruits, vegetables, lean proteins, and healthy fats. These foods are typically lower in calories and provide essential nutrients, which can support weight loss by promoting satiety and reducing overall calorie intake.

• Reduced Inflammation: AIP is designed to reduce inflammation, which is linked to obesity and metabolic disorders. By eliminating potentially inflammatory foods like gluten, dairy, and processed sugars, the diet may help individuals with underlying inflammation lose weight more effectively.

• Balanced Blood Sugar Levels: AIP promotes stable blood sugar levels by limiting refined carbohydrates and processed sugars. Balanced blood sugar levels can reduce cravings and overeating, making it easier to manage calorie intake.

• Elimination of Trigger Foods: The AIP diet involves an elimination phase where common food triggers, including grains, dairy, legumes, and nightshades, are removed. For individuals with sensitivities or allergies to these foods, their removal can lead to symptom relief and improved weight management.

• Gut Health: AIP emphasizes gut health, which is increasingly recognized as a factor in weight regulation. A healthy gut microbiome may support better digestion and nutrient absorption, potentially influencing weight.

• Reduced Processed Foods: The AIP diet discourages processed and convenience foods, which are often calorie-dense and nutrient-poor. By eliminating these foods, individuals may naturally consume fewer calories and lose weight.

• Elimination of Food Addictions: Some individuals have food sensitivities or addictions to certain foods that lead to overeating. The AIP elimination phase can break these cycles and promote healthier eating patterns.

It's important to note that weight loss results on the AIP diet can vary widely depending on individual factors, including starting weight, metabolic rate, adherence to the diet, and the presence of underlying health conditions. Additionally, not everyone who follows the AIP diet will experience weight loss; some individuals may maintain their current weight or experience weight gain.

Furthermore, the AIP diet should be approached primarily as a therapeutic dietary approach for managing autoimmune conditions and reducing inflammation. Weight loss, if it occurs, is often a secondary benefit.

Before starting the AIP diet or any weight loss program, it's advisable to consult with a healthcare professional or registered dietitian experienced in autoimmune conditions and weight management. They can provide guidance tailored to your specific health needs and goals.

AIP-compliant foods can aid in weight loss and help maintain a healthy weight due to several factors that promote a balanced and nutritious diet. Here's how these foods can support your weight loss and weight maintenance goals:

• Nutrient Density: AIP-compliant foods are predominantly whole, nutrient-dense options such as vegetables, lean proteins, fruits, and healthy fats. These foods are generally lower in calories but high in essential vitamins, minerals, and antioxidants, which support overall health and provide a sense of fullness without excessive calorie intake.

• Inflammation Reduction: The AIP diet eliminates many common inflammatory foods like gluten, dairy, processed sugars, and processed oils. Reducing inflammation can contribute to weight loss by addressing underlying metabolic and hormonal issues that can hinder weight management.

• Balanced Blood Sugar: AIP emphasizes whole foods and limits refined carbohydrates, added sugars, and processed snacks. This helps stabilize blood sugar levels, reducing the risk of energy crashes and sugar cravings that can lead to overeating.

• Improved Gut Health: The AIP diet encourages the consumption of foods that support gut health, such as bone broth, fermented foods, and fiber-rich vegetables. A healthy gut microbiome can enhance nutrient absorption, regulate appetite, and contribute to a balanced metabolism.

• Protein Emphasis: The diet places a strong emphasis on lean proteins like poultry, fish, and grass-fed meats. Protein is essential for muscle preservation and can promote satiety, helping to prevent muscle loss and hunger during weight loss.

• Fiber-Rich Foods: Many AIP-compliant vegetables and fruits are high in dietary fiber. Fiber contributes to feelings of fullness and helps regulate digestion, reducing the likelihood of overeating.

• Balanced Macronutrients: AIP encourages a balanced intake of macronutrients, including carbohydrates, proteins, and fats. This balance supports a sustainable eating pattern that provides energy and satisfies hunger.

• Minimized Processed Foods: Processed and convenience foods, often high in empty calories and unhealthy additives, are discouraged on the AIP diet. This helps individuals avoid calorie-dense, nutrient-poor options that contribute to weight gain.

• Individualized Approach: The AIP diet allows for individualization based on specific needs and tolerances. As you reintroduce foods during the transition phase, you can personalize your diet according to your body's unique responses, which can be conducive to long-term weight maintenance.

• Lifestyle Changes: Beyond diet, the AIP diet emphasizes lifestyle factors like stress management, adequate sleep, and regular physical activity, all of which play integral roles in weight management and overall well-being.

It's important to note that while AIP-compliant foods can provide a strong foundation for weight loss and maintenance, individual results may vary. Weight management is influenced by various factors, including genetics, activity level, and metabolic rate. Additionally, the AIP diet is primarily designed to address autoimmune conditions and inflammation, so it may not be suitable as a sole weight loss strategy for everyone.

Before embarking on any diet, including the AIP diet, it's advisable to consult with a healthcare provider or registered dietitian to ensure that your dietary choices align with your specific health goals and needs. They can provide personalized guidance and support on your weight loss and overall health journey.

DIFFICULTIES THAT PEOPLE MAY ENCOUNTER WHILE FOLLOWING THE AIP DIET

While the Autoimmune Protocol (AIP) diet can be highly effective in managing autoimmune conditions and improving overall health, it can also present challenges and difficulties for individuals. Here are some common difficulties that people may encounter while following the AIP diet:

1. Restrictiveness: The AIP diet is highly restrictive during the elimination phase, which can make it challenging to find a variety of foods to enjoy. The limited food choices can lead to feelings of deprivation and boredom.

2. Social Isolation: Eating out or socializing with friends and family can become more difficult due to the dietary restrictions of the AIP diet. Some individuals may feel isolated or left out in social settings.

3. Time-Consuming: Preparing AIP-compliant meals from scratch can be time-consuming, especially when compared to the convenience of processed and fast foods. This can be a barrier for individuals with busy lifestyles.

4. Expense: High-quality, organic, and pasture-raised foods, which are often recommended on the AIP diet, can be more expensive than conventional options. This can strain the budget for some individuals and families.

5. Learning Curve: Adhering to the AIP diet requires a significant amount of research and learning about which foods are allowed and which to avoid. It can take time to become familiar with the guidelines and identify AIP-friendly recipes.

6. Cravings: Eliminating certain foods, especially those that are comforting or culturally significant, can lead to cravings. Managing cravings for non-compliant foods can be challenging, especially in the early stages of the diet.

7. Limited Convenience Foods: Many convenience foods and snacks are off-limits on the AIP diet, making it difficult to find quick and easy options when you're on the go.

8. Meal Planning and Preparation: Planning and preparing AIP-compliant meals may require more effort and organization than individuals are used to. It can be difficult to consistently maintain this level of preparation.

9. Gut Healing: Some individuals may experience digestive discomfort as their gut heals during the AIP protocol. This can include symptoms like bloating, gas, or changes in bowel habits.

10. Emotional Impact: The AIP diet can have an emotional impact, especially if individuals are accustomed to using food for comfort or emotional reasons. Coping with stress and emotions without relying on certain foods can be challenging.

11. Reintroduction Phase: The reintroduction phase can also be challenging, as it involves systematically reintroducing foods that were previously eliminated to identify triggers. This requires patience and careful monitoring of symptoms.

12. Lack of Immediate Results: Some individuals may not experience immediate improvements in their symptoms or may find that the AIP diet doesn't resolve all their health issues. This can be discouraging for those seeking rapid relief.

It's important to acknowledge these difficulties and challenges associated with the AIP diet. However, many individuals have successfully overcome these obstacles by seeking support from healthcare professionals, dietitians, and AIP communities. Additionally, the long-term benefits of improved health and symptom management often outweigh the initial challenges of the diet for those with autoimmune conditions.

SUPPLEMENTS TO TAKE WHILE ON THE AIP DIET

While the Autoimmune Protocol (AIP) diet focuses primarily on nutrient-dense whole foods to support overall health and manage autoimmune conditions, some individuals may choose to supplement their diet to ensure they are meeting their nutritional needs. It's important to consult with a healthcare professional or registered dietitian experienced in the AIP diet to determine if supplements are necessary for your specific circumstances. Here are some supplements commonly considered while on the AIP diet:

• Digestive Enzymes: Digestive enzymes may be beneficial for individuals who experience digestive issues while on the AIP diet. They can aid in the digestion of fats, proteins, and carbohydrates, potentially reducing bloating and discomfort.

• Probiotics: Probiotic supplements can help support gut health by promoting the growth of beneficial gut bacteria. This can be particularly important for individuals with autoimmune conditions, as gut health is often a key factor.

• Fish Oil or Omega-3 Fatty Acids: Omega-3 fatty acids, found in fish oil supplements, can help reduce inflammation and support overall health. They may be especially useful if you're not consuming fatty fish regularly.

• Vitamin D: Many people, including those with autoimmune conditions, are deficient in vitamin D. A supplement can help maintain optimal levels, as vitamin D plays a crucial role in immune function.

• Multivitamin and Mineral Supplements: A high-quality multivitamin and mineral supplement can provide additional nutrients that may be lacking in your diet. Look for one without additives or non-compliant ingredients.

• Collagen Peptides: Collagen supplements may support gut health, joint health, and skin health. Collagen is often included in AIP-compliant protein sources, but some individuals choose to supplement it.

• L-Glutamine: L-Glutamine is an amino acid that may support gut healing. It can be considered if you have gastrointestinal issues.

• Zinc: Zinc is essential for immune function and may be beneficial for individuals with autoimmune conditions. However, it's important not to take excessive zinc, as it can interfere with the absorption of other minerals.

• Iron: Some individuals with autoimmune conditions, such as celiac disease, may be at risk of iron deficiency. Iron supplements should only be taken under the guidance of a healthcare professional and if a deficiency is confirmed.

• B Vitamins: A high-quality B-complex supplement can provide essential B vitamins. Ensure that it doesn't contain any non-compliant ingredients.

• Turmeric (Curcumin) Supplements: Turmeric supplements, particularly those containing curcumin, may help reduce inflammation. However, it's advisable to consult with a healthcare professional before adding these supplements.

• Herbal Supplements: Some herbal supplements, such as licorice root or slippery elm, may be used to support gut health. Consult with a healthcare professional for guidance.

Remember that supplements should not be used as a replacement for a well-balanced AIP-compliant diet. It's crucial to consult with a healthcare professional to assess your specific nutritional needs, determine which supplements may be appropriate for you, and establish the right dosages. Additionally, regular monitoring of nutrient levels through blood tests can help ensure that supplementation is tailored to your individual requirements.

LIFESTYLE FACTORS THAT SUPPORT WEIGHT LOSS

Lifestyle factors play a significant role in supporting weight loss and maintaining a healthy weight over the long term. When combined with a balanced diet, these factors can enhance your weight loss efforts and promote overall well-being. Here are key lifestyle factors that support weight loss:

1. Regular Physical Activity:

Engaging in regular exercise is essential for burning calories, improving metabolism, and building lean muscle mass. Aim for at least 150 minutes of moderate-intensity aerobic activity or 75 minutes of vigorous-intensity aerobic activity each week, along with strength training exercises on two or more days.

2. Balanced Diet:

A well-balanced and nutrient-dense diet is crucial for weight loss. Focus on whole foods, including lean proteins, fruits, vegetables, whole grains, and healthy fats. Avoid or limit processed and high-calorie foods.

3. Portion Control:

Be mindful of portion sizes. Overeating, even healthy foods, can lead to weight gain. Use smaller plates and utensils, and pay attention to hunger and fullness cues.

4. Regular Meal Timing:

Establish a regular eating schedule with consistent meal and snack times. This helps regulate hunger and prevents excessive calorie consumption.

5. Adequate Hydration:

Drinking enough water is vital for overall health and can help control appetite. Sometimes, thirst is mistaken for hunger, leading to unnecessary snacking.

6. Sleep Quality:

Aim for 7-9 hours of quality sleep per night. Inadequate sleep can disrupt hormones that regulate appetite and lead to weight gain.

7. Stress Management:

Chronic stress can trigger emotional eating and weight gain. Practice stress-reduction techniques such as meditation, yoga, deep breathing, or spending time in nature.

8. Mindful Eating:

Pay attention to what you eat and how you eat. Mindful eating involves savoring each bite, eating without distractions, and recognizing when you are full.

9. Social Support:

Surround yourself with a supportive social network. Share your weight loss goals with friends or family members who can encourage and motivate you.

10. Self-Monitoring:

Keep a food journal to track your meals, snacks, and emotional triggers for eating. Monitoring your progress can help identify areas for improvement.

11. Regular Physical Checkups:

Visit your healthcare provider for regular checkups and discuss your weight loss goals. They can provide guidance and monitor your overall health.

12. Gradual Changes:

Make gradual and sustainable changes to your diet and lifestyle. Extreme diets or rapid weight loss strategies are often unsustainable and can lead to weight regain.

13. Long-Term Perspective:

View weight loss as a long-term journey rather than a quick fix. Aim for sustainable lifestyle changes that you can maintain over time.

14. Education and Awareness:

Stay informed about nutrition and health. Understand the nutritional value of foods and make informed choices.

15. Positive Mindset:

Maintain a positive attitude and focus on the progress you've made, rather than fixating on setbacks. Weight loss can be challenging, but a positive mindset is essential for success.

Remember that everyone's weight loss journey is unique, and what works for one person may not work for another. It's essential to tailor these lifestyle factors to your individual needs and preferences. Consulting with a healthcare professional or registered dietitian can provide personalized guidance and support on your weight loss journey.

HOW TO SET REALISTIC WEIGHT LOSS GOALS

Setting realistic weight loss goals is crucial for achieving success and maintaining motivation on your weight loss journey. Unrealistic goals can lead to frustration and disappointment, while achievable goals can boost confidence and keep you on track. Here's a step-by-step guide on how to set realistic weight loss goals:

• Assess Your Current Situation:

Begin by evaluating your current weight, body composition, and overall health. Consider factors like age, gender, medical conditions, and fitness level.

• Define Your Motivation:

Identify why you want to lose weight. Your motivation can be health-related, such as managing a medical condition or reducing the risk of chronic diseases, or it may be for personal reasons like improving self-esteem or feeling more energetic.

• Consult with a Healthcare Professional:

If you have any medical conditions or concerns, consult with a healthcare provider or registered dietitian. They can help you determine a healthy and safe weight loss goal that considers your individual health needs.

• Understand Healthy Weight Loss Rates:

Realize that safe and sustainable weight loss typically ranges from 0.5 to 2 pounds per week. Rapid weight loss often leads to muscle loss and is harder to maintain.

• Set Specific Goals:

Define your weight loss goals in specific terms. For example, instead of saying "I want to lose weight," say "I want to lose 20 pounds in six months."

• Break Down Larger Goals:

If you have a significant amount of weight to lose, break your goal into smaller, more manageable milestones. Celebrating these mini-successes along the way can keep you motivated.

• Consider Non-Scale Goals:

Weight loss isn't the only measure of success. Consider setting non-scale goals, such as improving your fitness level, increasing energy, or fitting into a specific clothing size.

• Use the SMART Criteria:

a. Specific: Clearly define what you want to achieve.

b. Measurable: Determine how you'll measure your progress (e.g., pounds lost, inches lost).

c. Achievable: Ensure your goal is realistic given your circumstances.

d. Relevant: Align your goal with your motivation and values.

e. Time-Bound: Set a deadline for when you want to achieve your goal.

• Educate Yourself:

Learn about healthy eating, exercise, and sustainable lifestyle changes. Understanding the process can help you set more realistic goals.

• Seek Support:

Share your goals with friends, family, or a support group. Having a support system can provide encouragement and accountability.

• Track Your Progress:

Use a journal, app, or spreadsheet to track your progress. Regularly reviewing your achievements can help you stay on course.

• Be Flexible:

Be open to adjusting your goals as needed. Life can be unpredictable, and circumstances may change. It's okay to revise your goals to stay realistic.

• Focus on Health, Not Perfection:

Shift your focus from achieving a "perfect" body to improving your overall health and well-being. A healthy lifestyle should be sustainable and enjoyable.

• Celebrate Achievements:

Celebrate your successes, whether big or small. Recognize your hard work and determination along the way.

• Stay Patient and Persistent:

Understand that weight loss is a journey with ups and downs. Be patient with yourself and stay persistent even when faced with challenges.

Setting realistic weight loss goals is about finding a balance between ambition and practicality. With the right mindset, support, and a clear plan, you can work toward achieving your goals in a healthy and sustainable way.

IMPORTANCE OF THESE LIFESTYLE FACTORS IN WEIGHT LOSS

Lifestyle factors play a pivotal role in weight loss, as they significantly influence an individual's ability to shed excess pounds and maintain a healthy weight over the long term. Understanding the importance of these lifestyle factors is crucial for anyone embarking on a weight loss journey. Here are the key reasons why lifestyle factors are integral to weight loss success:

• Caloric Balance: Lifestyle factors directly impact the balance between calories consumed and calories expended. Weight loss occurs when you create a calorie deficit by consuming fewer calories than you burn through daily activities and exercise. A healthy lifestyle helps maintain this balance.

• Sustainable Behavior Change: Lifestyle factors focus on adopting sustainable changes in eating habits, physical activity, and overall wellness. These changes are more likely to be maintained over time, ensuring long-term weight management.

• Healthy Eating Habits: Lifestyle factors emphasize the importance of making nutritious food choices. Eating whole, nutrient-dense foods helps reduce calorie intake while ensuring that your body receives essential vitamins and minerals.

• Physical Activity: Regular physical activity is essential for burning calories, increasing metabolism, preserving muscle mass, and improving overall health. Lifestyle changes that prioritize exercise contribute to weight loss and overall fitness.

• Metabolic Health: Lifestyle factors can positively influence metabolic health, including insulin sensitivity and hormone regulation. Improved metabolic health can lead to more effective weight loss and better weight maintenance.

• Habit Formation: Lifestyle changes aim to establish healthy habits. Over time, these habits become ingrained and automatic, making it easier to maintain a healthy lifestyle and avoid weight regain.

• Stress Management: Chronic stress can lead to emotional eating and weight gain. Incorporating stress-reduction techniques such as mindfulness, meditation, and relaxation exercises can support weight loss efforts.

• Improved Sleep: Quality sleep is crucial for weight loss and overall well-being. A lack of sleep can disrupt hormones that regulate appetite and lead to increased calorie consumption.

• Social Support: Building a support network of friends, family, or a weight loss group can provide encouragement, accountability, and motivation during the weight loss journey.

• Mindful Eating: Lifestyle factors promote mindful eating practices, encouraging individuals to pay attention to hunger and fullness cues, savor their food, and make conscious food choices.

• Self-Efficacy: As individuals experience success with lifestyle changes, their confidence in their ability to achieve weight loss goals (self-efficacy) increases, further supporting their efforts.

• Health Improvements: Lifestyle changes often lead to improvements in overall health, including reductions in blood pressure, cholesterol levels, and the risk of chronic diseases. These health benefits are significant motivators for weight loss.

• Long-Term Success: Lifestyle factors are geared toward long-term success rather than quick fixes. A sustainable approach to weight loss is more likely to prevent weight regain.

• Mental Well-Being: A balanced lifestyle that includes regular exercise and healthy eating can positively impact mental health, reducing stress, anxiety, and symptoms of depression that may contribute to overeating.

• Body Composition: Lifestyle factors support the preservation of lean muscle mass during weight loss, which is essential for maintaining a healthy metabolism and achieving a favorable body composition.

In summary, lifestyle factors are fundamental to weight loss because they encompass sustainable changes in diet, physical activity, stress management, and overall well-being. By addressing these factors, individuals can increase their chances of achieving their weight loss goals and sustaining a healthier lifestyle in the long run.

TIPS FOR MEAL PLANNING, GROCERY SHOPPING AND KITCHEN PREPARATION

Meal planning, grocery shopping, and kitchen preparation are essential aspects of maintaining a healthy diet and lifestyle. Here are some tips to help you streamline these processes and make them more efficient:

Meal Planning:

• Set Clear Goals: Determine your dietary goals, whether it's weight loss, improving nutrition, or accommodating dietary restrictions. Your goals will guide your meal planning choices.

• Choose a Planning Schedule: Decide how often you'll plan your meals — weekly, bi-weekly, or monthly. A weekly plan is often a good starting point.

• Create a Meal Calendar: Use a calendar or meal planning app to map out your meals for the chosen period. Include breakfast, lunch, dinner, and snacks.

• Consider Leftovers: Plan for leftovers to minimize food waste. You can prepare larger portions and use them for subsequent meals.

• Balance Nutrients: Ensure your meal plan includes a balance of protein, carbohydrates, healthy fats, and a variety of fruits and vegetables. This promotes overall nutrition and satiety.

• Prep for Busy Days: Plan simpler meals or leftovers for days when you have limited time or energy to cook.

Grocery Shopping:

• Stick to Your List: Create a detailed shopping list based on your meal plan and stick to it. This helps you avoid impulse purchases.

• Shop the Perimeter: In most grocery stores, fresh produce, lean proteins, and dairy are located around the perimeter. Focus on these sections for healthier choices.

• Read Labels: When purchasing packaged foods, read labels carefully to check for added sugars, unhealthy fats, and artificial ingredients.

• Buy in Bulk (for Non-Perishables): Stock up on non-perishable staples like rice, quinoa, and canned goods to reduce the frequency of shopping trips.

• Choose Seasonal Produce: Seasonal fruits and vegetables are often fresher and more affordable. Incorporate them into your meal plan.

• Buy Frozen Foods: Frozen fruits, vegetables, and proteins can be a convenient and nutritious option, especially for items not in season.

• Avoid Shopping Hungry: Eat a meal or snack before going grocery shopping to avoid making impulsive, unhealthy choices.

Kitchen Preparation:

• Organize Your Kitchen: Keep your kitchen organized and tidy to make meal preparation more efficient. Know where your utensils, pots, and pans are located.

• Invest in Kitchen Tools: Invest in quality kitchen tools that make meal preparation easier, such as a good knife, cutting board, blender, and food processor.

• Prep Ingredients in Advance: Wash, chop, and portion fruits, vegetables, and proteins in advance. Store them in containers for easy access during meal prep.

• Batch Cooking: Cook larger quantities of grains, proteins, or sauces and freeze them in portions for quick, healthy meals on busy days.

• Plan for Leftovers: Cook extra portions during dinner for lunch the next day or freeze them for future meals.

• Use Cooking Shortcuts: Take advantage of time-saving products like pre-cut vegetables, canned beans, or rotisserie chicken for quick meals.

• Clean as You Go: Clean dishes and surfaces as you cook to minimize post-meal cleanup.

• Meal Prep Days: Designate specific days for meal prep, where you prepare multiple meals at once. This can save time during the week.

By incorporating these tips into your meal planning, grocery shopping, and kitchen preparation routines, you can make healthier eating more convenient and sustainable. Planning ahead and being organized in the kitchen can contribute to your overall success in maintaining a nutritious diet and achieving your health goals.

HOW TO MAINTAIN THE WEIGHT LOST USING THE AIP DIET

Maintaining weight loss achieved through the Autoimmune Protocol (AIP) diet, or any other weight loss method, requires ongoing commitment and a shift towards a sustainable, healthy lifestyle. Here are some strategies to help you maintain the weight you've lost while following the AIP diet:

• Stick to the Principles of AIP: Continue to prioritize AIP-compliant foods, focusing on whole, nutrient-dense options that support your overall health and well-being.

• Monitor Portion Sizes: Pay attention to portion sizes to prevent overeating. Be mindful of hunger and fullness cues, and avoid large, calorie-dense meals.

• Regular Physical Activity: Maintain a consistent exercise routine that includes a mix of cardiovascular, strength-training, and flexibility exercises. Regular physical activity is key to weight maintenance.

• Stay Hydrated: Drink plenty of water throughout the day. Sometimes, thirst is mistaken for hunger, leading to unnecessary calorie consumption.

• Meal Planning and Prep: Continue meal planning and preparation to ensure you have AIP-compliant foods readily available. This reduces the temptation to resort to unhealthy options when you're hungry.

• Mindful Eating: Practice mindful eating by savoring each bite, eating without distractions, and paying attention to the flavors and textures of your food. This can help you make conscious choices and prevent overeating.

• Regular Monitoring: Continue to track your meals, snacks, and progress, even after achieving your weight loss goals. Self-monitoring can help you stay accountable and recognize any potential issues early.

• Regular Check-Ins: Periodically consult with a healthcare professional or registered dietitian experienced in AIP to assess your dietary choices, address any concerns, and ensure you are meeting your nutritional needs.

• Be Prepared for Challenges: Recognize that maintaining weight loss may come with occasional challenges, such as social gatherings or stress. Plan ahead for these situations and have strategies in place to make healthy choices.

• Celebrate Non-Scale Victories: Shift your focus from the number on the scale to non-scale victories like increased energy, improved sleep, or physical fitness milestones. These achievements can be motivating and affirm your healthy habits.

• Avoid Extreme Dieting: Avoid extreme diets or drastic calorie restrictions, as they are often unsustainable and can lead to weight regain. Focus on a balanced and sustainable approach to eating.

• Stay Connected to Support Systems: Continue to engage with your support network, whether it's friends, family, or an AIP community. Sharing your experiences and challenges can provide valuable encouragement.

• Regular Health Checkups: Schedule regular checkups with your healthcare provider to monitor your overall health, including weight, blood pressure, and any relevant health markers.

• Adjust as Needed: Be open to adjusting your diet and exercise routines as your needs change. Factors like age, activity level, and metabolism can influence your dietary requirements.

• Mindset and Self-Care: Maintain a positive mindset and prioritize self-care practices, such as stress management, relaxation techniques, and sleep hygiene.

Remember that maintaining weight loss is a long-term commitment that involves continued dedication to a healthy lifestyle. While the AIP diet can be a valuable tool for weight loss and health improvement, it's essential to transition from a weight loss mindset to one focused on long-term well-being and sustainable habits.

Tracking the rate of weight loss is a helpful way to monitor your progress and adjust your approach as needed. Here are steps to effectively track the rate of weight loss:

1. Set Clear Goals:

Determine your weight loss goals, including the target amount of weight you want to lose and the timeframe in which you'd like to achieve it. Ensure your goals are specific, measurable, and realistic.

2. Use a Scale:

A bathroom scale is a straightforward tool for tracking your weight. Weigh yourself consistently, preferably at the same time of day and under similar conditions (e.g., after waking up and using the restroom). Record your weight in a journal or a digital tracking app.

3. Document Your Progress:

Create a weight loss journal or use a digital app to record your weight regularly. Tracking your weight over time allows you to identify trends and patterns.

4. Choose a Consistent Tracking Schedule:

Decide on the frequency of tracking that works for you, whether it's daily, weekly, or bi-weekly. Consistency is key to accurate tracking.

5. Track Other Metrics:

In addition to weight, consider tracking other metrics like body measurements (waist, hips, chest), body fat percentage, and even photographs. These can provide a more comprehensive view of your progress.

6. Calculate Your Rate of Weight Loss:

To calculate your rate of weight loss, subtract your current weight from your starting weight, and then divide by the number of weeks or months it took to lose that weight. For example, if you lost 10 pounds over 2 months, your rate of weight loss would be 5 pounds per month.

7. Analyze Trends:

Don't get discouraged by day-to-day fluctuations in weight, as these are common. Instead, focus on the overall trend over several weeks or months. Look for consistent patterns of weight loss or maintenance.

8. Set Realistic Expectations:

Keep in mind that weight loss rates can vary from person to person. A safe and sustainable rate of weight loss is typically 0.5 to 2 pounds per week. Rapid weight loss may not be healthy or sustainable.

9. Adjust Your Approach:

Regularly assess your progress and be willing to adjust your dietary and exercise habits as needed. If you're not progressing at the desired rate, consider consulting a healthcare provider or registered dietitian for guidance.

10. Focus on Non-Scale Victories:

While tracking weight is important, also celebrate non-scale victories like improved energy, better sleep, and clothing fitting more comfortably. These achievements can be just as meaningful.

11. Stay Patient and Persistent:

Weight loss can be a slow and nonlinear process. It's essential to stay patient and persistent, especially during plateaus or periods of slower progress.

12. Seek Support:

Share your progress with friends, family, or a support group. Accountability and encouragement from others can be motivating.

Remember that weight loss is just one aspect of improving your overall health. It's essential to focus on adopting a sustainable, balanced lifestyle that includes a healthy diet, regular physical activity, and stress management. The rate of weight loss may vary, but consistency in healthy habits will lead to long-term success.

TIPS FOR NAVIGATING SOCIAL EVENTS, DINING OUT, AND TRAVELING WHILE ON THE AIP DIET.

Navigating social events, dining out, and traveling while following the Autoimmune Protocol (AIP) diet can present challenges, but with some preparation and strategies, you can maintain your dietary restrictions and still enjoy these experiences. Here are some tips for successfully managing AIP in social settings:

1. Plan Ahead:

• Research Restaurants: When dining out, research restaurants in advance. Look for those that offer AIP-friendly options or are willing to accommodate dietary restrictions. Many restaurants now have their menus available online, which can help you make informed choices.

• Pack Snacks: Bring AIP-compliant snacks with you when traveling or attending social events. Having your snacks on hand ensures you won't go hungry if there are limited AIP options available.

2. Communicate Clearly:

• Notify Hosts or Servers: If you're attending a social event or dining out, communicate your dietary needs to the host or server in advance. They may be able to make accommodations or provide you with information about AIP-friendly menu items.

- Ask Questions: Don't hesitate to ask questions about ingredients and preparation methods. Servers and chefs are usually willing to assist with dietary restrictions when asked politely.

3. BYO (Bring Your Own):

- Bring Your Own Dish: If you're attending a potluck or social gathering, consider bringing an AIP-friendly dish that you can enjoy and share with others.

- Travel with AIP Staples: When traveling, carry AIP staples like coconut oil, AIP-approved snacks, and herbal tea bags. These items can be used to supplement your meals if you have limited food options.

4. Learn to Modify:

- Modify Menu Items: Look for menu items that can be easily modified to fit your AIP requirements. For example, ask for salads without nightshades or dressings with AIP-friendly ingredients.

- Customize Your Order: Don't be afraid to customize your order to meet your needs. Most restaurants are willing to accommodate substitutions and adjustments.

5. Stay Informed:

• Stay Informed About Local Cuisine: If you're traveling to a new destination, research the local cuisine and ingredients commonly used. This can help you anticipate AIP-friendly options and avoid potential pitfalls.

• Learn About Hidden Ingredients: Be aware of hidden ingredients that may not be obvious. For example, some spice blends and sauces may contain non-compliant ingredients.

6. Be Patient and Flexible:

• Stay Patient: Understand that it may take some time to find suitable options or educate others about your dietary needs. Be patient with yourself and those around you.

• Flexibility: While it's essential to adhere to the AIP diet, allow yourself some flexibility when traveling or in social settings. Focus on the best possible choices given the circumstances.

7. Have a Go-To List of Safe Foods:

• Safe Foods List: Maintain a list of AIP-compliant foods and ingredients that you can refer to when dining out or shopping for groceries in unfamiliar places.

8. Consider Intermittent Fasting:

• Intermittent Fasting: Some individuals on the AIP diet find intermittent fasting helpful when traveling or attending social events. Fasting during certain hours of the day can simplify meal planning and reduce the need to find AIP-compliant food.

Remember that with practice and experience, navigating social events, dining out, and traveling while on the AIP diet becomes more manageable. Being prepared, communicating your needs, and having a positive attitude are key to successfully enjoying these experiences while maintaining your dietary restrictions.

THE IMPORTANCE OF KEEPING A FOOD DIARY AND SYMPTOM JOURNAL.

Keeping a food diary and symptom journal can be invaluable tools when following a specialized diet like the Autoimmune Protocol (AIP) or managing any dietary-related health condition. Here's why they are important:

1. Identifying Food Triggers:

• Food Allergies and Sensitivities: A food diary helps you pinpoint specific foods that may trigger allergies or sensitivities. By tracking what you eat and any subsequent symptoms, you can establish connections between certain foods and adverse reactions.

• AIP Compliance: For those on the AIP diet, it's crucial to ensure strict compliance to identify any potential triggers accurately. A food diary helps you stay accountable and avoid accidental consumption of non-compliant foods.

2. Personalizing Your Diet:

• Individual Variability: Everyone's tolerance to specific foods can vary. What works for one person on the AIP diet may not work for another. Keeping a food diary allows you to tailor your diet to your unique needs and responses.

• Identifying Safe Foods: Over time, a food diary helps you create a list of safe and well-tolerated foods. This list can be a valuable resource when planning meals and snacks.

3. Tracking Symptoms:

• Symptom Management: A symptom journal allows you to track the severity and frequency of symptoms related to your condition. This can be crucial for managing autoimmune diseases or other health conditions effectively.

• Identifying Patterns: By recording symptoms alongside your food intake, you can identify patterns and potential triggers. This insight can help you and your healthcare provider make more informed decisions about dietary modifications or treatments.

4. Monitoring Progress:

• Assessing Improvement: Over time, a food diary and symptom journal enable you to gauge your progress. You can see whether your symptoms are improving, worsening, or remaining stable, which can inform your healthcare decisions.

• Identifying Setbacks: In some cases, you may experience setbacks or flare-ups. A journal helps you identify the possible causes and adjust your diet or treatment accordingly.

5. Guiding Reintroductions:

• AIP Reintroduction: For those on the AIP diet, a food diary is essential when reintroducing eliminated foods. It helps you track reactions to specific foods during the reintroduction phase and determine which foods can be safely reintroduced and which should remain excluded.

6. Facilitating Healthcare Discussions:

• Effective Communication: When you visit healthcare providers or dietitians, having a detailed food diary and symptom journal provides them with valuable information. It allows for more informed discussions about your condition and dietary management.

• Treatment Adjustments: Healthcare professionals can use your journal to make recommendations, adjustments to your treatment plan, or further diagnostic tests based on your dietary and symptom history.

7. Promoting Accountability:

• Compliance: Maintaining a food diary encourages adherence to your dietary plan. It holds you accountable for your food choices, making it less likely that you'll deviate from your prescribed diet.

8. Reducing Uncertainty and Anxiety:

• Empowerment: Keeping track of what you eat and how it affects you empowers you to take control of your health. It reduces the uncertainty and anxiety often associated with managing dietary conditions.

9. Supporting Research and Documentation:

• Data for Research: If you participate in clinical research related to your condition or diet, a well-kept food diary and symptom journal can serve as valuable data for researchers and contribute to advancements in understanding and treatment.

In summary, a food diary and symptom journal are essential tools for managing dietary conditions, identifying food triggers, and personalizing your diet. They provide a clear record of your dietary choices, symptoms, and progress, making it easier to work with healthcare providers and make informed decisions about your health and well-being.

CHAPTER TWO

Sweet Potato Hash with Ground Turkey

Ingredients:

• 1 sweet potato, diced

• 1/2 pound ground turkey

• 1 onion, diced

• 1 garlic clove, minced

• 1 tsp coconut oil

• Salt and pepper (omit pepper for AIP)

Instructions:

1. Heat coconut oil in a skillet over medium heat.

2. Add onions and garlic and sauté until softened.

3. Add ground turkey and sweet potatoes, and cook until turkey is browned and sweet potatoes are tender.

4. Season with salt to taste.

AIP Breakfast Bowl

Ingredients:

- 1 baked sweet potato, mashed

- 1/2 cup cooked ground beef or turkey

- 1/2 cup cooked greens (e.g., spinach or kale)

- 1/2 avocado, sliced

Instructions:

1. Combine mashed sweet potato, cooked meat, and greens in a bowl.

2. Top with sliced avocado and season with salt.

Coconut Flour Pancakes

Ingredients:

- 1/4 cup coconut flour

- 2 eggs

- 1/4 cup coconut milk

- 1/2 tsp baking soda

- 1/4 tsp cream of tartar

- Pinch of salt

Instructions:

1. Mix all ingredients in a bowl until a smooth batter forms.

2. Heat a skillet over medium heat and grease with coconut oil.

3. Pour small portions of the batter onto the skillet and cook until bubbles form, then flip and cook until golden brown.

AIP Smoothie Bowl

Ingredients:

- 1/2 cup frozen mixed berries

- 1/2 ripe banana

- 1/2 cup coconut milk

- 1 tbsp coconut oil

- Toppings: sliced kiwi, shredded coconut, and chopped mango

Instructions:

1. Blend the frozen berries, banana, coconut milk, and coconut oil until smooth.

2. Pour the smoothie into a bowl and top with sliced kiwi, shredded coconut, and chopped mango.

Baked Acorn Squash with Sausage

Ingredients:

- 1 acorn squash, halved and seeds removed

- 1/2 pound AIP-compliant sausage

- 1/2 onion, diced

- 1 tsp coconut oil

- Salt and fresh herbs (e.g., sage or thyme)

Instructions:

1. Preheat the oven to 375°F (190°C).

2. Rub the inside of the acorn squash with coconut oil and season with salt.

3. In a skillet, cook the sausage and onions until browned.

4. Stuff the acorn squash halves with the sausage mixture and bake for about 45 minutes, until squash is tender.

AIP Breakfast Soup

Ingredients:

• 1 cup bone broth

• 1 cup cooked chicken, shredded

• 1 cup cauliflower florets

• 1/2 cup carrots, diced

• 1/2 cup zucchini, diced

• Fresh parsley for garnish

Instructions:

1. In a pot, combine bone broth, chicken, cauliflower, carrots, and zucchini.

2. Simmer until vegetables are tender. Garnish with fresh parsley before serving.

Cauliflower and Bacon Breakfast Bowl

Ingredients:

- 2 cups cauliflower rice

- 4 slices AIP-compliant bacon, cooked and crumbled

- 1/4 cup green onions, chopped

- 1/4 cup sautéed spinach

Instructions:

1. Sauté cauliflower rice until tender.

2. Top with crumbled bacon, green onions, and sautéed spinach.

Tuna Salad Stuffed Avocado

Ingredients:

- 1 ripe avocado, halved and pitted

- 1 can of AIP-compliant tuna, drained

- 1/4 cup diced cucumber

- 1/4 cup diced red bell pepper

- 1 tbsp olive oil

- Lemon juice, salt, and fresh herbs (e.g., cilantro or parsley) for seasoning

Instructions:

1. In a bowl, combine tuna, cucumber, red bell pepper, olive oil, and lemon juice.

2. Season with salt and fresh herbs. Spoon the tuna salad into the avocado halves.

AIP Breakfast Sausage Patties

Ingredients:

- 1 pound ground pork

- 1/2 tsp dried sage

- 1/2 tsp dried thyme

- 1/2 tsp garlic powder

- Salt to taste

Instructions:

1. Mix all ingredients in a bowl.

2. Form the mixture into small sausage patties.

3. Cook in a skillet over medium heat until browned and cooked through.

Baked Plantain Frittata

Ingredients:

- 2 ripe plantains, sliced

- 6 eggs

- 1/2 cup coconut milk

- 1 cup cooked spinach

- 1/2 onion, diced

- 1 tsp coconut oil

- Salt and fresh herbs for seasoning

Instructions:

1. Preheat the oven to 350°F (175°C).

2. In an oven-safe skillet, sauté onions in coconut oil until translucent. Add sliced plantains and cook until lightly browned.

3. In a bowl, whisk together eggs, coconut milk, cooked spinach, salt, and fresh herbs.

4. Pour the egg mixture over the plantains and onions in the skillet.

5. Bake in the oven for 20-25 minutes, until the frittata is set and slightly golden on top.

AIP Breakfast Casserole

Ingredients:

• 1 pound ground turkey

• 1 cup diced sweet potatoes

• 1/2 cup diced carrots

- 1/2 cup diced zucchini

- 1/2 cup diced bell peppers

- 1/2 onion, diced

- 6 eggs

- 1/4 cup coconut milk

- Salt and herbs (e.g., basil or oregano) for seasoning

Instructions:

1. Preheat the oven to 350°F (175°C).

2. In a skillet, cook the ground turkey until browned, then set aside. Sauté the diced vegetables until tender.

3. In a bowl, whisk together eggs, coconut milk, salt, and herbs.

4. Grease a baking dish, layer the cooked turkey and sautéed vegetables, and pour the egg mixture over them.

5. Bake for 25-30 minutes until the casserole is set.

Ingredients:

- 2 medium zucchinis, spiralized into noodles

- 1/4 cup AIP-friendly pesto sauce

- Chopped fresh basil for garnish

Instructions:

1. Sauté the zucchini noodles in a pan until tender.

2. Toss with AIP pesto sauce. Garnish with chopped fresh basil.

Chicken and Vegetable Stir-Fry

Ingredients:

- 1 cup cooked chicken, diced

- 1 cup broccoli florets

- 1/2 cup sliced mushrooms

- 1/2 cup sliced carrots

- 1/2 onion, sliced

- 2 tbsp coconut aminos

- 1 tsp coconut oil

- Salt and garlic powder for seasoning

Instructions:

1. In a skillet, sauté onions and carrots in coconut oil until slightly softened.

2. Add broccoli, mushrooms, cooked chicken, and coconut aminos.

3. Stir-fry until the vegetables are tender and the chicken is heated through.

AIP Breakfast Soup with Ground Beef

Ingredients:

- 1 cup bone broth

- 1/2 cup cooked ground beef

- 1/2 cup chopped spinach

- 1/2 cup chopped butternut squash

- 1/2 tsp dried rosemary

- Salt and fresh parsley for garnish

Instructions:

1. Simmer bone broth, ground beef, spinach, and butternut squash until the vegetables are tender.

2. Season with dried rosemary and salt.

3. Garnish with fresh parsley before serving.

AIP Avocado and Mango Smoothie

Ingredients:

- 1 ripe avocado

- 1/2 cup chopped mango

- 1/2 cup coconut milk

- 1/2 cup water

- 1 tsp honey (optional, omit if preferred)

Instructions:

1. Blend avocado, mango, coconut milk, water, and honey (if using) until smooth.

Baked Apples with Cinnamon

Ingredients:

- 2 apples, cored and halved

- 1 tsp cinnamon

- 1 tbsp coconut oil

Instructions:

1. Preheat the oven to 350°F (175°C).

2. Place the apple halves on a baking sheet. Sprinkle with cinnamon and dot with coconut oil.

3. Bake for about 20-25 minutes until the apples are soft and slightly caramelized.

AIP Plantain Waffles

Ingredients:

- 2 ripe plantains

- 2 tbsp coconut flour

- 2 eggs

- 1/2 tsp baking soda

- Pinch of salt

Instructions:

1. Blend plantains, coconut flour, eggs, baking soda, and salt until smooth.

2. Preheat a waffle iron and cook the batter according to the manufacturer's instructions.

AIP Breakfast Skillet with Ground Bison

Ingredients:

- 1/2 pound ground bison

- 1 sweet potato, diced

- 1/2 onion, diced

- 1/2 cup sliced Brussels sprouts

- 1/4 cup chopped parsley

- 1 tsp coconut oil

- Salt and fresh thyme for seasoning

Instructions:

1. In a skillet, cook the ground bison until browned, then set aside.

2. Sauté sweet potatoes, onions, and Brussels sprouts in coconut oil until tender.

3. Add the cooked bison back to the skillet, season with salt and fresh thyme, and garnish with chopped parsley.

AIP Breakfast Meatballs

Ingredients:

- 1 pound ground pork

- 1/2 cup chopped spinach

- 1/4 cup chopped green onions

- 1/4 cup chopped fresh cilantro

- 1/2 tsp garlic powder

- Salt and dried basil for seasoning

Instructions:

1. Preheat the oven to 375°F (190°C).

2. Mix ground pork, chopped spinach, green onions, cilantro, garlic powder, salt, and dried basil in a bowl.

3. Form the mixture into small meatballs and place them on a baking sheet.

4. Bake for 20-25 minutes or until cooked through.

AIP Porridge with Banana and Coconut

Ingredients:

- 2 ripe bananas, mashed

- 1/2 cup coconut flour

- 1/2 cup coconut milk

- 1/2 tsp cinnamon

- 1/4 tsp vanilla extract (AIP-compliant)

- Shredded coconut and sliced bananas for topping

Instructions:

1. Mix mashed bananas, coconut flour, coconut milk, cinnamon, and vanilla extract in a bowl until smooth.

2. Serve in a bowl and top with shredded coconut and sliced bananas.

AIP Chicken and Vegetable Stir-Fry

Ingredients:

• 1 pound boneless, skinless chicken thighs, thinly sliced

• 2 cups broccoli florets

• 1 cup sliced carrots

• 1/2 cup sliced zucchini

• 1/2 onion, sliced

• 2 tbsp coconut aminos

• 1 tbsp coconut oil

• Salt and ginger (omit for AIP) for seasoning

Instructions:

1. Heat coconut oil in a large skillet over medium-high heat.

2. Add sliced chicken and sauté until no longer pink. Add vegetables and continue to stir-fry until they are tender.

3. Season with coconut aminos, salt, and ginger (if tolerated).

AIP Tuna Salad Lettuce Wraps

Ingredients:

• 2 cans of AIP-compliant tuna, drained

• 1/4 cup finely diced celery

• 1/4 cup diced cucumber

• 1/4 cup diced red bell pepper

• 2 tbsp olive oil

• Lemon juice, salt, and fresh herbs (e.g., basil or parsley) for seasoning

• Large lettuce leaves for wrapping

Instructions:

1. In a bowl, combine drained tuna, celery, cucumber, red bell pepper, olive oil, and lemon juice.

2. Season with salt and fresh herbs.

3. Spoon the tuna salad into lettuce leaves to make wraps.

AIP Butternut Squash Soup

Ingredients:

• 1 small butternut squash, peeled and diced

• 1 onion, chopped

• 2 cups bone broth

• 1/2 cup coconut milk

• 1 tsp coconut oil

• 1/2 tsp dried thyme

• Salt and fresh chives for garnish

Instructions:

1. In a large pot, heat coconut oil over medium heat.

2. Add chopped onion and sauté until translucent.

3. Add diced butternut squash, bone broth, and dried thyme. Bring to a boil, then reduce heat and simmer until squash is tender.

4. Puree the soup with an immersion blender, stir in coconut milk, and season with salt.

5. Garnish with fresh chives before serving.

AIP Zucchini Noodles with Avocado Pesto

Ingredients:

• 2 medium zucchinis, spiralized into noodles

• 1 ripe avocado

• 1/4 cup fresh basil leaves

• 2 cloves garlic (omit for AIP)

• 2 tbsp olive oil

• Lemon juice, salt, and pepper (omit pepper for AIP) for seasoning

Instructions:

1. In a blender or food processor, combine avocado, basil, garlic (if tolerated), olive oil, and lemon juice. Blend until smooth.

2. Sauté zucchini noodles in a pan until tender.

3. Toss the noodles with the avocado pesto and season with salt.

AIP Turkey and Avocado Lettuce Wraps

Ingredients:

• 1/2 pound ground turkey

• 1/2 avocado, diced

• 1/4 cup diced cucumber

• 1/4 cup diced red onion

• 2 tbsp olive oil

• Lemon juice, salt, and fresh cilantro for seasoning

• Large lettuce leaves for wrapping

Instructions:

1. In a skillet, cook ground turkey until browned.

2. In a bowl, combine diced avocado, cucumber, red onion, olive oil, lemon juice, salt, and fresh cilantro.

3. Spoon the turkey mixture into lettuce leaves to make wraps.

AIP Salmon Salad with Lemon Herb Dressing

Ingredients:

• 2 cups cooked salmon, flaked

• 2 cups mixed salad greens

• 1/4 cup diced cucumber

• 1/4 cup diced red bell pepper

• 1/4 cup sliced radishes

• 1/4 cup chopped fresh dill

• 2 tbsp olive oil

• Lemon juice, salt, and fresh chives for dressing

Instructions:

1. In a large bowl, combine flaked salmon, salad greens, cucumber, red bell pepper, radishes, and fresh dill.

2. Drizzle with olive oil and lemon juice, and season with salt.

3. Garnish with fresh chives.

AIP Cabbage Rolls with Ground Beef

Ingredients:

• 1 head of cabbage

• 1/2-pound ground beef

• 1/2 onion, diced

• 1 cup cauliflower rice

• 1 cup AIP-compliant tomato sauce

• 1 tsp dried oregano

• Salt and fresh parsley for garnish

Instructions:

1. Preheat the oven to 350°F (175°C).

2. Remove cabbage leaves and blanch them in boiling water until pliable.

3. In a skillet, cook ground beef and onions until browned.

4. Mix in cauliflower rice, dried oregano, and half of the AIP-compliant tomato sauce. Fill cabbage leaves with the beef mixture, roll them up, and place in a baking dish.

5. Pour the remaining tomato sauce over the rolls and bake for 30 minutes. Garnish with fresh parsley before serving.

AIP Shrimp and Avocado Salad

Ingredients:

• 1 cup cooked shrimp, peeled and deveined

• 1/2 avocado, diced

• 1/2 cup sliced cucumber

• 1/4 cup sliced red onion

• 2 tbsp olive oil

• Lemon juice, salt, and fresh parsley for dressing

Instructions:

1. In a bowl, combine cooked shrimp, diced avocado, sliced cucumber, and red onion.

2. Drizzle with olive oil, lemon juice, and season with salt.

3. Garnish with fresh parsley.

AIP Turkey and Sweet Potato Hash

Ingredients:

• 1/2-pound ground turkey

• 1 sweet potato, diced

• 1/2 onion, diced

• 1/2 cup sliced green beans

• 1 tbsp coconut oil

• Salt and fresh thyme for seasoning

Instructions:

1. Heat coconut oil in a skillet over medium heat.

2. Add diced sweet potato and cook until tender. Push sweet potato to one side and add ground turkey to the skillet, cooking until browned.

3. Add diced onion and sliced green beans, and sauté until vegetables are tender.

4. Season with salt and fresh thyme.

AIP Roasted Veggie Salad

Ingredients:

• 2 cups mixed roasted vegetables (e.g., carrots, beets, and asparagus)

• 2 cups mixed salad greens

• 1/4 cup sliced radishes

• 2 tbsp olive oil

• Balsamic vinegar, salt, and fresh basil for dressing

Instructions:

1. Toss roasted vegetables, salad greens, and sliced radishes in a bowl.

2. Drizzle with olive oil, balsamic vinegar, and season with salt.

3. Garnish with fresh basil.

AIP Chicken and Avocado Salad

Ingredients:

• 1 cup cooked chicken, shredded

• 1/2 avocado, diced

• 1/4 cup diced cucumber

• 1/4 cup diced jicama

• 2 tbsp olive oil

• Lemon juice, salt, and fresh mint for dressing

Instructions:

1. In a bowl, combine shredded chicken, diced avocado, cucumber, and jicama.

2. Drizzle with olive oil, lemon juice, and season with salt.

3. Garnish with fresh mint.

AIP Beef and Vegetable Soup

Ingredients:

• 1/2-pound ground beef

• 2 cups chopped carrots

• 1 cup chopped celery

• 1 cup chopped zucchini

• 1/2 onion, diced

• 4 cups bone broth

• 1 tsp dried rosemary

• Salt and fresh parsley for garnish

Instructions:

1. In a pot, brown ground beef and diced onions.

2. Add chopped carrots, celery, zucchini, bone broth, dried rosemary, and salt. Simmer until vegetables are tender.

3. Garnish with fresh parsley before serving.

AIP Roasted Beet and Citrus Salad

Ingredients:

• 2 roasted beets, sliced

• 1 orange, segmented

• 1/4 cup pomegranate seeds

• 2 tbsp olive oil

• Lemon juice, salt, and fresh basil for dressing

Instructions:

1. Arrange sliced roasted beets and orange segments on a plate.

2. Sprinkle with pomegranate seeds.

3. Drizzle with olive oil, lemon juice, and season with salt. Garnish with fresh basil.

AIP Turkey and Cranberry Salad

Ingredients:

1. 1 cup cooked turkey, diced

2. 1/4 cup fresh cranberries

3. 1/4 cup diced celery

4. 1/4 cup chopped green apples

5. 2 tbsp olive oil

6. Lemon juice, salt, and fresh parsley for dressing

Instructions:

1. In a bowl, combine diced turkey, fresh cranberries, diced celery, and chopped green apples.

2. Drizzle with olive oil, lemon juice, and season with salt.

3. Garnish with fresh parsley.

AIP Baked Acorn Squash with Ground Pork

Ingredients:

- 1 acorn squash, halved and seeded

- 1/2-pound ground pork

- 1/2 cup diced butternut squash

- 1/2 cup diced onions

- 1 tsp coconut oil

- Cinnamon, salt, and fresh sage for seasoning

Instructions:

1. Preheat the oven to 375°F (190°C).

2. Rub the inside of the acorn squash with coconut oil and season with cinnamon and salt.

3. In a skillet, brown ground pork and diced onions. Fill acorn squash halves with the pork mixture and add diced butternut squash.

4. Bake for about 45 minutes or until the squash is tender. Garnish with fresh sage.

AIP Beef and Broccoli Stir-Fry

Ingredients:

- 1 pound thinly sliced beef

- 2 cups broccoli florets

- 1/2 cup sliced bell peppers

- 1/2 cup sliced mushrooms

- 1/2 onion, sliced

- 2 tbsp coconut aminos

- 1 tbsp coconut oil

- Salt and ginger (omit for AIP) for seasoning

Instructions:

1. In a skillet, heat coconut oil over medium-high heat.

2. Add sliced beef and cook until no longer pink. Remove from the skillet. Sauté broccoli, bell peppers, mushrooms, and onions until tender.

3. Return the cooked beef to the skillet and stir in coconut aminos, salt, and ginger (if tolerated).

AIP Cucumber and Radish Salad

Ingredients:

• 2 cups sliced cucumbers

• 1 cup sliced radishes

• 1/4 cup sliced red onion

• 2 tbsp olive oil

• Apple cider vinegar, salt, and fresh dill for dressing

Instructions:

1. In a bowl, combine sliced cucumbers, radishes, and red onion.

2. Drizzle with olive oil, apple cider vinegar, and season with salt.

3. Garnish with fresh dill.

AIP Chicken and Spinach Soup

Ingredients:

• 1 cup cooked chicken, shredded

• 2 cups chopped spinach

• 1/2 cup diced carrots

• 1/2 cup diced zucchini

• 1/2 onion, diced

• 4 cups bone broth

• 1 tsp dried thyme

• Salt and fresh parsley for garnish

Instructions:

1. In a pot, combine shredded chicken, chopped spinach, diced carrots, diced zucchini, diced onion, bone broth, dried thyme, and salt.

2. Simmer until vegetables are tender.

3. Garnish with fresh parsley before serving.

AIP Spaghetti Squash with Bolognese Sauce

Ingredients:

• 1 spaghetti squash, halved and seeded

• 1/2 pound ground beef

• 1/2 cup diced carrots

• 1/2 cup diced celery

• 1/2 cup diced onions

• 2 cups AIP-compliant tomato sauce

• 1 tsp dried basil

• Salt and fresh basil for garnish

Instructions:

1. Preheat the oven to 375°F (190°C).

2. Place the spaghetti squash halves cut side down on a baking sheet and roast for about 45 minutes or until tender.

3. In a skillet, brown ground beef and diced onions.

4. Add diced carrots, diced celery, AIP-compliant tomato sauce, dried basil, and salt. Simmer until vegetables are tender.

5. Scrape the spaghetti squash flesh with a fork to create "noodles" and top with Bolognese sauce. Garnish with fresh basil.

AIP Chicken and Asparagus Salad

Ingredients:

• 1 cup cooked chicken, diced

• 2 cups steamed asparagus, chopped

• 1/2 cup diced cucumber

• 1/4 cup sliced green onions

• 2 tbsp olive oil

• Lemon juice, salt, and fresh tarragon for dressing

Instructions:

1. In a bowl, combine diced chicken, chopped asparagus, diced cucumber, and sliced green onions.

2. Drizzle with olive oil, lemon juice, and season with salt.

3. Garnish with fresh tarragon.

AIP Lemon Herb Baked Chicken

Ingredients:

- 4 bone-in, skin-on chicken thighs

- 2 tbsp olive oil

- Juice of 1 lemon

- 2 cloves garlic (omit for AIP)

- 1 tsp dried thyme

- Salt and fresh parsley for garnish

Instructions:

1. Preheat the oven to 375°F (190°C).

2. In a bowl, whisk together olive oil, lemon juice, minced garlic (if tolerated), dried thyme, and a pinch of salt.

3. Place chicken thighs in a baking dish, pour the lemon herb mixture over them, and bake for 30-35 minutes or until cooked through.

4. Garnish with fresh parsley before serving.

AIP Salmon with Roasted Vegetables

Ingredients:

• 2 salmon fillets

• 2 cups mixed roasted vegetables (e.g., sweet potatoes, carrots, and broccoli)

• 2 tbsp olive oil

• Lemon juice, salt, and fresh dill for seasoning

Instructions:

1. Preheat the oven to 375°F (190°C).

2. Brush salmon fillets with olive oil and season with lemon juice, salt, and fresh dill.

3. Place the salmon fillets on a baking sheet and roast for 15-20 minutes or until the salmon flakes easily.

4. Serve with mixed roasted vegetables.

AIP Salmon with Roasted Vegetables

AIP Beef and Vegetable Skillet

Ingredients:

• 1 pound ground beef

• 2 cups diced butternut squash

• 1 cup sliced green beans

• 1/2 onion, diced

• 2 tbsp coconut oil

• Salt and dried rosemary for seasoning

Instructions:

1. In a skillet, brown ground beef and diced onions in coconut oil.

2. Add diced butternut squash and sliced green beans. Sauté until vegetables are tender.

3. Season with salt and dried rosemary.

AIP Zucchini Noodles with Pesto and Shrimp

Ingredients:

* 2 medium zucchinis, spiralized into noodles

* 1 cup fresh basil leaves

* 2 cloves garlic (omit for AIP)

* 1/4 cup olive oil

* 1/2-pound cooked shrimp, peeled and deveined

* Lemon juice, salt, and fresh parsley for seasoning

Instructions:

1. In a blender or food processor, combine basil, garlic (if tolerated), and olive oil. Blend until smooth.

2. Sauté zucchini noodles in a pan until tender. Toss the noodles with pesto and cooked shrimp.

3. Season with lemon juice, salt, and garnish with fresh parsley.

AIP Pork and Pineapple Stir-Fry

Ingredients:

* 1 pound pork tenderloin, thinly sliced

- 1 cup diced pineapple

- 1/2 cup sliced bell peppers

- 1/2 cup sliced mushrooms

- 1/2 onion, sliced

- 2 tbsp coconut aminos

- 1 tbsp coconut oil

- Salt and ginger (omit for AIP) for seasoning

Instructions:

1. In a skillet, heat coconut oil over medium-high heat.

2. Add sliced pork and cook until browned. Add diced pineapple, sliced bell peppers, sliced mushrooms, and sliced onions.

3. Stir in coconut aminos and season with salt and ginger (if tolerated).

AIP Turkey and Sweet Potato Casserole

Ingredients:

- 1 pound ground turkey

- 2 cups diced sweet potatoes

- 1/2 cup diced onions

- 1/2 cup diced carrots

- 1/2 cup AIP-compliant tomato sauce

- 1 tsp dried thyme

- Salt and fresh parsley for garnish

Instructions:

1. Preheat the oven to 375°F (190°C).

2. In a skillet, brown ground turkey and diced onions.

3. Add diced sweet potatoes, diced carrots, AIP-compliant tomato sauce, dried thyme, and a pinch of salt.

4. Transfer the mixture to a baking dish, cover with foil, and bake for 30-35 minutes or until sweet potatoes are tender.

5. Garnish with fresh parsley before serving.

Ingredients:

- 1/2-pound shrimp, peeled and deveined

- 2 cups broccoli florets

- 2 cloves garlic (omit for AIP)

- Juice of 1 lemon

- 2 tbsp olive oil

- Salt and fresh parsley for seasoning

Instructions:

1. In a skillet, heat olive oil over medium-high heat.

2. Add peeled shrimp and cook until pink and opaque. Add broccoli florets and minced garlic (if tolerated).

3. Squeeze lemon juice over the shrimp and broccoli. Season with salt and garnish with fresh parsley.

AIP Baked Cod with Lemon and Herbs

Ingredients:

- 2 cod fillets

- Juice of 1 lemon

- 2 tbsp olive oil

- 1 tsp dried thyme

- Salt and fresh dill for seasoning

Instructions:

1. Preheat the oven to 375°F (190°C).

2. Place cod fillets on a baking sheet. Drizzle with olive oil, lemon juice, and sprinkle with dried thyme and salt.

3. Bake for 15-20 minutes or until the cod flakes easily. Garnish with fresh dill before serving.

AIP Turkey and Vegetable Stir-Fry

Ingredients:

- 1/2-pound ground turkey

- 2 cups mixed vegetables (e.g., snow peas, carrots, and bell peppers)

- 1/2 onion, sliced

- 2 tbsp coconut aminos

- 1 tbsp coconut oil

- Salt and ginger (omit for AIP) for seasoning

Instructions:

1. In a skillet, heat coconut oil over medium-high heat.

2. Brown ground turkey and sliced onions. Add mixed vegetables and stir-fry until tender.

3. Season with coconut aminos, salt, and ginger (if tolerated).

AIP Beef and Cabbage Rolls

Ingredients:

- 1 head of cabbage

- 1/2-pound ground beef

- 1/2 cup cauliflower rice

- 1/2 cup diced carrots

- 1/2 cup diced onions

- 2 cups AIP-compliant tomato sauce

- 1 tsp dried oregano

- Salt and fresh parsley for garnish

Instructions:

1. Preheat the oven to 350°F (175°C).

2. Remove cabbage leaves and blanch them in boiling water until pliable.

3. In a skillet, brown ground beef and diced onions. Mix in cauliflower rice, diced carrots, AIP-compliant tomato sauce, dried oregano, and a pinch of salt.

4. Fill cabbage leaves with the beef mixture, roll them up, and place in a baking dish.

5. Pour the remaining tomato sauce over the rolls and bake for 30 minutes.

6. Garnish with fresh parsley before serving.

AIP Garlic and Herb Roasted Chicken

Ingredients:

- 1 whole chicken (3-4 pounds)

- 2 tbsp olive oil

- 2 cloves garlic (omit for AIP)

- 1 tsp dried rosemary

- 1 tsp dried thyme

- Salt and fresh parsley for garnish

Instructions:

1. Preheat the oven to 375°F (190°C).

2. In a small bowl, mix olive oil, minced garlic (if tolerated), dried rosemary, dried thyme, and a pinch of salt.

3. Rub the mixture all over the chicken. Place the chicken in a roasting pan and roast for approximately 1 hour or until the chicken is cooked through.

4. Garnish with fresh parsley before serving.

Ingredients:

• 1 spaghetti squash, halved and seeded

• 2 cups fresh basil leaves

• 2 cloves garlic (omit for AIP)

• 1/4 cup olive oil

• Lemon juice, salt, and fresh basil for seasoning

Instructions:

1. Preheat the oven to 375°F (190°C).

2. Place the spaghetti squash halves cut side down on a baking sheet and roast for about 45 minutes or until tender.

3. In a blender or food processor, combine fresh basil, minced garlic (if tolerated), olive oil, and lemon juice. Blend until smooth.

4. Scrape the spaghetti squash flesh with a fork to create "noodles" and toss with the AIP pesto.

5. Season with salt and garnish with fresh basil.

AIP Thai-Inspired Shrimp Soup

Ingredients:

• 1/2-pound cooked shrimp, peeled and deveined

• 2 cups sliced zucchini

• 1/2 cup sliced carrots

• 1/2 cup sliced bell peppers

• 1/2 onion, sliced

• 2 cups bone broth

• 1/4 cup coconut milk

• 1 tsp ginger (omit for AIP)

• Salt and fresh cilantro for garnish

Instructions:

1. In a pot, combine sliced zucchini, sliced carrots, sliced bell peppers, sliced onions, bone broth, and ginger (if tolerated).

2. Simmer until vegetables are tender.

3. Stir in cooked shrimp and coconut milk, and heat until shrimp are warmed.

4. Season with salt and garnish with fresh cilantro.

AIP Baked Turkey Meatballs

Ingredients:

• 1 pound ground turkey

• 1/4 cup chopped fresh parsley

• 1/4 cup diced green onions

• 1/4 cup diced carrots

• 1/4 cup diced zucchini

• 1/4 cup coconut flour

• 1 tsp garlic powder

• Salt and dried basil for seasoning

Instructions:

1. Preheat the oven to 375°F (190°C).

2. In a bowl, combine ground turkey, chopped parsley, diced green onions, diced carrots, diced zucchini, coconut flour, garlic powder, salt, and dried basil.

3. Form the mixture into small meatballs and place them on a baking sheet.

4. Bake for 20-25 minutes or until cooked through.

AIP Beef and Broccoli Casserole

Ingredients:

• 1 pound ground beef

• 2 cups chopped broccoli florets

• 1/2 cup sliced mushrooms

• 1/2 cup diced onions

• 1/2 cup AIP-compliant tomato sauce

• 1 tsp dried oregano

• Salt and fresh basil for garnish

Instructions:

1. Preheat the oven to 375°F (190°C).

2. In a skillet, brown ground beef and diced onions.

3. Add chopped broccoli florets, sliced mushrooms, AIP-compliant tomato sauce, dried oregano, and a pinch of salt.

4. Transfer the mixture to a baking dish and bake for 30-35 minutes or until the broccoli is tender.

5. Garnish with fresh basil before serving.

AIP Lemon Herb Grilled Shrimp

Ingredients:

- 1/2 pound large shrimp, peeled and deveined

- 2 tbsp olive oil

- Juice of 1 lemon

- 2 cloves garlic (omit for AIP)

- 1 tsp dried basil

• Salt and fresh chives for garnish

Instructions:

1. In a bowl, whisk together olive oil, lemon juice, minced garlic (if tolerated), dried basil, and a pinch of salt.

2. Thread shrimp onto skewers. Brush the shrimp with the lemon herb mixture.

3. Grill the shrimp over medium-high heat for 2-3 minutes per side or until they turn pink.

4. Garnish with fresh chives before serving.

AIP Coconut Curry Chicken

Ingredients:

• 4 boneless, skinless chicken thighs

• 1 cup diced sweet potatoes

• 1/2 cup diced onions

• 1/2 cup sliced bell peppers

• 1/2 cup sliced zucchini

- 1 can (13.5 oz) coconut milk

- 2 tbsp curry powder (AIP-compliant)

- Salt and fresh cilantro for garnish

Instructions:

1. In a skillet, brown chicken thighs over medium-high heat. Remove from the skillet and set aside.

2. In the same skillet, sauté diced sweet potatoes, diced onions, sliced bell peppers, and sliced zucchini until tender.

3. Stir in coconut milk and curry powder. Return the cooked chicken to the skillet and simmer until chicken is cooked through.

4. Season with salt and garnish with fresh cilantro.

AIP Turkey and Vegetable Soup

Ingredients:

- 1/2-pound ground turkey

- 2 cups mixed vegetables (e.g., carrots, celery, and green beans)

- 1/2 onion, diced

- 4 cups bone broth

- 1 tsp dried thyme

- Salt and fresh parsley for garnish

Instructions:

1. In a pot, brown ground turkey and diced onions.

2. Add mixed vegetables and bone broth. Simmer until vegetables are tender.

3. Season with dried thyme, salt, and garnish with fresh parsley.

AIP Lemon Garlic Roasted Shrimp and Vegetables

Ingredients:

- 1/2-pound large shrimp, peeled and deveined

- 2 cups mixed roasted vegetables (e.g., carrots, Brussels sprouts, and asparagus)

- 2 tbsp olive oil

- Juice of 1 lemon

- 2 cloves garlic (omit for AIP)

- Salt and fresh thyme for seasoning

Instructions:

1. Preheat the oven to 375°F (190°C).

2. Toss mixed vegetables with olive oil, lemon juice, minced garlic (if tolerated), and fresh thyme. Roast the vegetables for 20-25 minutes or until tender.

3. In the last 5 minutes of roasting, add the shrimp and cook until pink and opaque.

4. Season with salt before serving.

AIP Shepherd's Pie

Ingredients:

- 1 pound ground beef

- 1 cup mashed sweet potatoes

- 1/2 cup diced carrots

- 1/2 cup diced onions

- 1/2 cup diced celery

- 1/2 cup bone broth

- 1 tsp dried thyme

- Salt and fresh parsley for garnish

Instructions:

1. In a skillet, brown ground beef, diced onions, diced celery, and diced carrots.

2. Stir in bone broth and dried thyme. Simmer until the mixture thickens.

3. Transfer the beef mixture to a baking dish. Spread mashed sweet potatoes on top.

4. Bake at 375°F (190°C) for 20-25 minutes or until the top is golden.

5. Garnish with fresh parsley before serving.

CONCLUSION

In conclusion, the Autoimmune Protocol (AIP) diet offers a valuable framework not only for managing autoimmune conditions and reducing inflammation but also for supporting weight loss and maintaining a healthy weight. By focusing on whole, nutrient-dense foods, reducing inflammation, and promoting a balanced eating pattern, AIP-compliant foods can aid in weight loss and help keep it off.

The AIP diet's emphasis on whole foods, inflammation reduction, and gut health aligns with principles that support sustainable weight management. By choosing foods that nourish the body and minimize inflammation, individuals following the AIP diet may experience improvements in overall health and well-being, along with their weight loss goals.

It's important to remember that weight management is a complex and individualized journey, and the AIP diet should be approached with a focus on long-term health and well-being rather than solely as a weight loss strategy. Consulting with healthcare professionals or registered dietitians who specialize in autoimmune conditions and weight management is advisable to ensure that the AIP diet aligns with your specific health needs and goals.

Ultimately, the AIP diet serves as a valuable tool that, when used mindfully and personalized to individual preferences and tolerances, can contribute to achieving and maintaining a healthy weight while supporting overall health and vitality.

9 7 9 8 8 6 6 2 8 3 8 4 2